# JOHN ITNOYAH

# Save Yourself Now

*A Quick Guide on How to Easily Overcome Pain And Disease Affordably When Your Doctor Has Given Up And Left You to Suffer Or Die*

# Contents

# 1

# Introduction

This book is about what I have experienced and researched in life. It is not intended for use as a medical or legal reference. I am not a Doctor, nor do I claim to have medical expertise. I have the utmost respect for members of the medical profession.

However, at times it seems that these days there is greater concern for profit than for the care of their patients. In my lifetime Doctors have told me on two occasions that I would die within a matter of months. Interestingly the second time was nine years after the first death sentence and for a different problem. I am providing information for educational and entertainment purposes. Hopefully it will help you solve your problems.

Every human being is different, act accordingly on your own individual circumstances. What works for one might not work for others. Use common sense, moderation and caution in all things regarding your health. It is ok to be skeptical, however many times I have encountered people who demand to see peer reviewed research and hold it up as their gold standard for belief.Unfortunately the peer review process has been exposed as corrupt.

Science, E. O. G. (2020, October 28). *Fake peer-reviewing*. The Embassy of Good Science. https://embassy.science/wiki/Theme:Fb1a2e2a-aa2 a-4eb4-ac9c-c9567c2b401b


Thomas, S. P. (2018). Current controversies regarding peer review in scholarly journals. *Issues in Mental Health Nursing, 39*(2), 99–101. https://doi.org/10.1080/01612840.2018.1431443


It is good to be skeptical, but don't allow it to close your mind and hold you back from a healthy pain-free life.

# 2

# Cancer

Cancer is the number one cause of death in the world. Some say heart disease is number one, but does it really matter? Your doctor has just diagnosed you with cancer and depending on which of the more than 200 types of cancer you have he will give you an estimated time of your eventual demise. And then says he can treat you with:

- Chemotherapy $1000 to $12,000 monthly
- Radiation $9,000 monthly
- Immunotherapy $10,000 to $12,500 monthly
- Surgery Varies on circumstances.

Your doctor will not tell you these costs up front.Nor will he tell you immediately that Chemotherapy and Radiation will damage your immune system. Immunotherapy is the last choice he will offer you usually after the first two have failed.

As an example of costs, last year I was unfortunately in the hospital for 10 days. The final cost was $318,000. Imagine you are in the hospital, get treated and then the monthly treatment costs begin to accumulate. The typical employer health insurance has a co-payment probably at about 25 percent. So, unless you are a millionaire or have really great health insurance cancer will put you into severe debt or bankrupt you if you survive.

Selby, K., RN. (2023, December 20). *High cost of cancer treatment: chemotherapy & other options.* Mesothelioma Center - Vital Services for Cancer Patients & Families. https://www.asbestos.com/featured-stories/high-cost-of-cancer-treatment/

On top of all of that it turns out that the conventional treatments do not work. There is no increase in survivability rate after treatment.Literally it's the same as if you did not get treated.

Faarfm, K. C. D. F. (2023, February 6). Some truths behind conventional cancer therapies. *Conners Clinic | Alternative Cancer Coaching.* https://www.connersclinic.com/the-truth-behind-conventional-cancer-therapies/

Also, cancer is primarily a failure of your immune system to remove damaged cells. Cells that continuously divide forming tumors and can spread to all parts of your body. Yet these treatments will damage or destroy your remaining immune system. Don't think surgery is a guaranteed life saver. If the surgeon misses a few cells the cancer is not gone. All of these therapies will fail and you will relapse if all the cancer cells are not removed. Relapse is almost certain if what caused your cancer is still within you.

You must eliminate the source of your cancer.

What causes cancer? This is a short, generalized list:

- Parasites, Microbes
- Toxins
- Forever Chemicals or PFAS
- DNA damage
- Spike proteins
- Poor diet

3

# Parasites, Microbes

arasites are organisms that live in you and feed on your tissues. They are detrimental and provide no benefits to the host. These include tapeworms, pinworms, roundworms to name just a few. Some of these are visible to the naked eye literally inches long. Here are some methods to remove parasites and other biologicals:

- Fenbendazole
- Ivermectin
- Hydrogen Peroxide
- Parasite cleanse

**Fenbendazole**

This starts with the Joe Tippens story. Joe Tippens was diagnosed with terminal lung cancer which then metastasized to all the other organs of his body. His Doctor told him he had three months to live. On a visit to a veterinarian friend to treat his dog. He was told about Fenbendazole which is usually used as an animal dewormer.

In drug studies involving mice the mice are usually dewormed with Fenbendazole before the drug trial starts. This is to ensure that there are no other factors that can skew the results of the trials. Several researchers noticed that some of the mice that had tumors were now tumor free after the treatment. One of these researchers then developed cancer and used Fenbendazole on herself. Within twelve weeks her glioblastoma had disappeared.

With nothing to lose Joe purchased the inexpensive dewormer and treated himself with a cocktail of Fenbendazole (222mg) with the addition of Curcumin (600mg) Vitamin E (800IU), CBD oil (25mg), Berberine and Quercetin. This is now known as the Joe Tippens Protocol. Three and a half months later he went back to the doctor and was declared cancer free. As of this date he is still cancer free.

*Get busy living.* (n.d.). https://mycancerstory.rocks/

## Ivermectin

Let me tell you the story of Danny L. Danny L. grew up on a farm. One day he left work, his drive home was about 35 miles. On the way home he experienced intense dizziness. Luckily as he tells it, it was nighttime, and he was able to focus on the side of the road.He stopped to get gas and fell out of the truck at the gas station. Got gas and went home and fell into bed. He was still dizzy when he woke up, so called in sick and went to the hospital.

After many tests he was diagnosed with vertigo and prescribed meclizine. Three weeks of bed rest later his dizziness never went away. Went to another doctor for a 2nd opinion. This one, an ear and throat specialist told him he was misdiagnosed as vertigo goes away in 15 hours. An MRI showed lesions on the brain. He was prescribed prednisone and amoxicillin. This drug cocktail gave him bad diarrhea. He then started experiencing what he describes as muddy memory, where he literally would forget what he was doing after he did it. A third doctor examined him and discovered bruises on his body.One bruise on his back covered half of his back. He was diagnosed with spirochetes, Parkinson's and Dementia.

He went to the hospital where they inserted a tube up his arm into his heart. This was to deliver a drug as close to his heart as possible. His prescriptions, including the IV drip, amounted to over 100 pills a day. He was assigned a home care nurse that visited once a week to check his blood and vital signs. This went on for 4 years 5 months and was told three times that he was going to die. Eventually his organs started failing.

One day he couldn't afford the latest prescription which was about 400 dollars and bought Equimax mistaking one of the ingredients in Equimax for the prescription drug. This cost him 12 dollars. Equimax is a drug for horses and states on it "Not for Human Consumption." The next morning after taking Equimax he was covered in sweat and felt better. Over the next several weeks whenever he felt bad, he repurchased Equimax. He did not know anything about dosages at that time and was basically experimenting on himself. In the third month he took a whole tube of Equimax. He was still doing the IV and 100 pills a day all throughout this time. By the 5th month he told the nurse to take the tube out of his heart. She was stunned and checked his medical history. It showed a massive improvement.

By this time all his friends and family had seen what he had gone through. From a weak dying man back to almost full health. One of his neighbors approached him about his 11-year-old daughter. She had a bad case of rheumatoid arthritis. Try Ivermectin, he was told and within days she was perfectly healthy. These encounters about health issues started to balloon.

Then Covid came and the negative comments about Ivermectin infuriated him. One woman asked him about her husband who was in the hospital with Covid. He told her to put ivermectin in water bottles and give them to him. She did and his oxygen level, which was at 60, went to 93 overnight.

Danny finally went back to the Doctor and did a full battery of tests. Three weeks later when the results came back the doctor was stunned and said he was clear as a bell. Heart enzymes which were at 29 percent were now 4 percent this meant that before he had a 29 percent chance of a heart attack, and this was now reduced to a 4 percent chance. All the tests were like that. All his internal organs had regenerated.

He then started a channel on Telegram which now has over 140 thousand members, many of whom relate their personal stories of curing their ailments. Including Cancer and Multiple Sclerosis. Ivermectin does not kill the parasite eggs in your body, so you must stop and restart the Protocol every few days to get them after they hatch. You can find Danny's life story and simple protocol of Ivermectin and lemon juice and distilled water here:

*Dirt road discussions.* (n.d.). Telegram. https://t.me/DirtRoadDiscussion/6895

**Hydrogen Peroxide**

Oxygen is the most essential element required for life. You can live without food for days, even weeks and months. Without water for days. But without Oxygen your lifespan is now measured in minutes. As it turns out the harmful bacteria and viruses in your body are anaerobic.

Meaning they live without Oxygen and in fact cannot survive in a highly oxygenated environment. Think about that fact, AIDs, Cancer, ulcers, Covid, Flu. The list is endless. Cancer tumors shrink in a highly oxygenated environment. In fact, cells can become cancerous in an oxygen deprived environment. Breathing Oxygen is not enough to highly oxygenate your body. It is estimated that only 15 percent of the Oxygen you breathe is utilized. You can oxygenate your drinking water by bubbling ozone through it but an ozonator costs up to $600.00. However, Food Grade Hydrogen Peroxide cost from 14 cents to $1.25 an ounce.

Hydrogen Peroxide at high concentrations is very dangerous. It will burn your skin on contact. It must be diluted in Distilled water. The recommended dose is 3 drops of 35% Food Grade Hydrogen Peroxide in 8 ounces of distilled water three times a day. You can increase the number of drops per day as days pass. Take on an empty stomach one hour before eating or three hours afterwards. For the complete Protocol and explanation of the use of Hydrogen Peroxide I highly recommend the book by Madison Cavanaugh. The One-Minute Cure for more details on Hydrogen Peroxide.

**Parasite Cleanse**

Here is a very simple and cheap cleanse. Mix Apple cider vinegar, clay, Epsom salts and baking soda in a tub of hot water and soak your feet. Get your cell phone to document the parasites visible to the naked eye. More complex and expensive cleanses involve Herbal remedies. These herbs include wormwood, clove and black walnut. A detailed Herbal cleanse can be found here:

*Parasite cleanse: DIY protocol, pills, and home remedy.* (n.d.). The Berkeley Well-Being Institute. https://www.berkeleywellbeing.com/parasite-cleanse-protocol-pills-home-remedy.html

## Herxheimer Reaction

After taking these healing solutions you might find yourself reacting poorly, headaches, body aches, sweating, nausea, chills and flu like symptoms.This is fine. This is a normal reaction to the toxins released by the dying parasites and other invasive organisms. This is not a negative sign; it is in fact a sign that the treatment is working. Drink lots of distilled water with a pinch of Celtic Sea salt to flush out the toxins.The salt is just to add minerals to the distilled water. The important thing is to not stop whatever Protocol you are using. More on this topic can be found here:

Phillips, K. (2020, July 27). Herxheimer reaction - Feeling worse before feeling better. *Colloidal Silver | Silver Colloids*. https://www.silver-collo ids.com/herxheimer-reaction/

# 4

# Toxins

Notice that every reference to drinking water refers to distilled water. This is because in most cases your tap water has been treated with chemicals such as Chlorine and Fluoride. Chlorine has been shown to damage your DNA. Studies on swimmers in chlorinated pools show an increase in the incidents of bladder cancer. Let's not forget your shower, immediately start using a shower filter that removes chlorine and fluoride. Chlorine uptake into your body is very fast; it takes only seconds.

Yeager, A. (2011, November 15). *A sip or quick dip could change your DNA - Research Blog*. Research Blog. https://researchblog.duke.edu/2011/11/15/a-sip-or-quick-dip-could-change-your-dna/

Fluoride is a chemical waste product. In the 1940s a major chemical company was being sued by local communities for their dumping of fluoride near their towns.That company created a massive publicity drive that touted the health benefits of Fluoride as a tooth enamel protector. They then sold off their waste product for a large profit. This deception was so successful that even today your dentist will admonish you to use fluoridated toothpaste and drink fluoridated water.

Boiling water does not remove Fluoride, it concentrates it in the water.
Fluoride is in your tap water, beverages made with fluoridated water, toothpaste and many other products. Tea is a hyperaccumulator of fluoride. The green tea you are so fond of contains fluoride. What many do not realize is that fluoride causes Dental Fluorosis (destruction of teeth enamel), Cognitive failure, Cardiac failure, Bone cancer, low IQ the list goes on and on. For a more complete list go here:

Miaomt, J. K. D. (2023). Fluoride exposure and human health risks. *IAOMT*. https://iaomt.org/resources/fluoride-facts/fluoride-exposur e-human-health-risks/

## Glyphosate

Glyphosate is the most widely used herbicide in the world.It is present on most of the foods you eat. It works by blocking the production of tyrosine, tryptophan and Phenylalanine. It kills most plants; it does not target specific plants. It decreases protein production. In humans and animals, it produces neurotoxic effects, mitochondrial dysfunction, behavioral and motor disorders. A more detailed description of the effects can be seen here:

Costas-Ferreira, C., Durán, R., & Faro, L. (2022). Toxic effects of glyphosate on the nervous system: a systematic review. *International Journal of Molecular Sciences, 23*(9), 4605. https://doi.org/10.3390/ ijms23094605

Many lawsuits have been filed against Monsanto, the now defunct company that produced Glyphosate. Millions of dollars have been awarded in settlements. If you have used Roundup and now have non-Hodgkin's lymphoma go here to see your lawsuit options:

Gaines, M. (2024, February 2). Roundup lawsuit update February 2024. *Forbes Advisor*. https://www.forbes.com/advisor/legal/product-liability/roundup-lawsuit-update/

The products that contain Glyphosate are too numerous to completely list. They include:

- Cookies
- Granola
- Water
- Orange juice
- Ice Cream
- Tampons
- Clothing

Luckily skin is difficult for Glyphosate to penetrate.Your goal is to avoid ingestion.For a more complete list of products go here:

Team, S. L. (2024, February 6). *Are you snacking on Cancer-Causing weed killer? Here are the foods you need to avoid.* Sokolove Law. https://www.sokolovelaw.com/blog/foods-glyphosate-cancer/

Drink distilled water. Many people have the belief that distilled water is bad for you that it is dead water and washes out your minerals. Distilled water will remove the toxins from your body. You can remineralize distilled water with a pinch of Celtic Sea Salt. I suggest Celtic Sea Salt because 90 percent of salt from China like the Himalayan pink salts have been shown to contain heavy metals like mercury due to their lax regulations on mining the salt.

## Chlormequat

This chemical, a pesticide, has been linked to heart disease, developmental and reproductive problems such as infertility and reducing fetal growth. It has been detected in 80 percent of people tested. It has been found in 92 percent of Oat based products such as Quaker Oats and Cheerios.

Research on the dangers of this pesticide is limited. Considering the damage done by another agricultural chemical Glyphosate caution should be taken. The good news is that Chlormequat leaves the body after 24 hours, however since testing shows it is still in the body this means there is continuous ingestion. In tests of food only 2 of 7 organic foods tested positive compared to 92 percent of non-organic food.

*EWG finds little-known toxic chemical in four out of five people tested.* (2024, February 15). Environmental Working Group. https://www.ewg.org/news-insights/news/2024/02/ewg-finds-little-known-toxic-chemical-four-out-five-people-tested

5

# Detox

A very simple and effective detox is to take 3 - 4 lbs of baking soda and put it into a tub of hot water. Soak in the tub until the water cools.

## Activated Charcoal

Activated charcoal binds to metal ions, it attaches to heavy metals and also beneficial minerals so make sure to supplement minerals three hours after ingestion. It also binds to positively charged particles such as pathogens and plastic.

## Bentonite Clay

Bentonite clay is also negatively charged like activated charcoal but has minerals and other nutrients. It can help repair your gut.

## Chlorella and Spirula

Chlorella, a green algae, removes heavy metals, Dioxin, BPs and other plastics. It is a great source of protein and minerals.Spirulina is a blue-green algae, it is similar to Chlorella is not as good in detox but is a better source of protein.

Calcium D-Glucarate

Supports the glucuronidation detoxification process which takes place in the liver and removes PCBs.

6

# Forever Chemicals (PFAS)

PFAS (short for per- and poly-fluoroalkyl substances) are made with highly toxic fluorinated chemicals. These chemicals are made up of Carbon and Fluorine atoms. Products that claim to be non-stick, stain-resistant, oil-resistant, flame-retardant and water-repellant are made from these PFAS chemicals. These chemicals do not break down in the environment and accumulate in our bodies for years. Very small quantities can induce cancers such as kidney, liver, pancreatic and testicular cancer. Other diseases include ulcerative colitis and thyroid disease.

*C8 Science Panel website.* (n.d.). http://www.c8sciencepanel.org/

In 1946 Dupont introduced Teflon. Yes that's right it's the non-stick coating on your frying pan. 3M took over the manufacture of Teflon and introduced Scotchgard. Gore-Tex is also a forever chemical. Every piece of clothing labeled water repellent contains PFAS chemicals. Fire fighter foam contains PFAS. PFAS has contaminated the entire world and has been discovered in drinking water. The cardboard and paper used for your fast food like burgers, popcorn bags, pizza and bakery bread is coated with PFAS chemicals.Paper bags, paper cups, paper plates and the plastic wrapping on food contains PFAS chemicals. The paper straw you use instead of a plastic straw contains PFAS. Whereas the plastic straw has no PFAS the paper straw tests positive for 21 different PFAS chemicals.

Timshina, A., Aristizabal-Henao, J. J., Da Silva, B. F., & Bowden, J. A. (2021). The last straw: Characterization of per- and polyfluoroalkyl substances in commercially-available plant-based drinking straws. *Chemosphere, 277,* 130238. https://doi.org/10.1016/j.chemosphere.2021.130238

It is an unfortunate fact that PFAS chemicals are everywhere.

What can you do to eliminate PFAS?

1. Buy foods and items labeled PFAS-free or PFOA-free
2. Drink distilled water or water filtered with a high quality filter
3. Educate yourself on PFAS contaminated areas and products. https://greensciencepolicy.org/our-work/pfas/
4. Detox yourself, use a combination of beta-glucan, vitamin C, and resveratrol. Beta-Glucans are "polysaccharides" that exist in whole foods, such as seaweed, grains, yeasts, mushrooms. Beta-Glucans from Bakers Yeast have long been used to boost the immune system.

7

# DNA Damage

It has now been revealed that the Covid vaccines by Pfizer and Moderna contain foreign DNA. The amount is in the billions of fragments per dose. Even more problematic is the discovery of Simian Virus 40 (SV40) in the vaccine which enables the integration of the DNA into the cells. This could impact the genes that turn a cell cancerous.

*Florida State Surgeon General calls for halt in the use of COVID-19 mRNA vaccines | Florida Department of Health.* (2024, January 20). https://www.floridahealth.gov/newsroom/2024/01/20240103-halt-use-covid19-mrna-vaccines.pr.html

Unfortunately most of us have taken the vaccine and the only solution now is not to take the boosters. Definitely do not take the so called 2 in 1 flu and covid booster. The last time I took a flu shot I got sick with the flu 3 days after the shot and it was the worst flu I ever had lasting for 6 months.

The history of vaccines is extremely problematic.There is controversy concerning the origin of the Spanish flu of 1918. Some say it actually originated from a vaccine administered to American soldiers.

*Did a vaccine experiment on US soldiers cause the 'Spanish flu'? - LewRockwell.* (2020, March 30). LewRockwell. https://www.lewrockwell.com/2020/03/no_author/did-a-vaccine-experiment-on-u-s-soldiers-cause-the-spanish-flu/

Despite continuous denials by the CDC and other institutional agencies the link between autism and vaccines continues to appear.The current rate of autism is approximately 1 in 36 and just over twenty years ago it was 1 in 250 children. Go back even further and autism is almost unknown and then they started vaccinating babies. The correlation is damning.

Wilson, R. (2023, September 1). *Childhood Vaccines cause Autism: The evidence and the institutional cover-up.* The Expose. https://expose-news.com/2023/09/01/childhood-vaccines-cause-autism-the-evidence-and-the-institutional-cover-up/

## Frequencies

What can repair DNA damage? This now touches on frequencies. Certain frequencies can affect your body and state of mind. Your cells are responsive to frequencies. The effect of frequencies have been known since ancient times.

Bells were known to have healing effects. In Russia it was well known that the plague avoided areas where the bells sounded. The unfortunate thing is that almost all the bells in the West have been destroyed. Pictures show thousands of bells in the past being melted down. The reasons for this destruction are varied.One is that the metal was utilized to make weapons for wars. Another hints at a wider, more malign goal where the beginning pharmaceutical industry did not want healing to be so widespread and easily available at no cost. Bells in Asia and Eastern regions still exist and those bells are still used for healing.

Admin, Admin, & Admin. (2021, December 6). *Influence of church bells on human health*. Orthodox Christian Tools/Store/Blog- Best Answers to Your Spiritual Questions - Answers to Your Spiritual Health Questions! https://orthochristiantools.com/influence-of-church-bells-on-huma n-health/

At this time we can duplicate the healing frequencies with modern equipment. The healing frequencies are now known. The one for DNA repair is 528hz also known as Divine Love.

Raccioppi, R. M. (2014, March 10). 528Hz - DNA repair - art and science of restorative frequencies. *Nyack-Piermont, NY Patch*. https://pa tch.com/new-york/nyack/528hz---dna-repair---art-and-science-of-restorative-frequencies

There are several tones known to have effects. These are known as the solfeggio frequencies.

- 174 Hz Pain relief
- 285 Hz regeneration
- 396 Hz freedom from fear, guilt and anxiety
- 417 Hz enable change and help
- 432 Hz calm and sleep

- 528 Hz DNA repair and miracles, increase cell life
- 639 Hz relationships, harmony, communication
- 741 Hz solutions, creativity, cleansing
- 852 Hz spirituality, intuition, inner strength, positivity
- 963 HZ oneness and unity

You can download these frequencies for free at:
https://www.tunepocket.com/solfeggio-frequencies/

**Royal Rife**

Dr Raymond Royal Rife (1888-1971) in 1933 invented a microscope he called a universal microscope which had a magnification of 60,000 diameters. Standard optical microscopes had a maximum magnification of 2500 diameters.

He used his microscope to see living viruses, he was the first person to accomplish this feat. The electron microscope can only view dead viruses. He then discovered the cancer microbe. He also discovered he could destroy viruses by resonance. Rife found the particular electromagnetic frequency of the virus or bacteria and then used an impulse of the same frequency to destroy it. He called this the "Mortal Oscillatory Rate.".

In 1934, an experiment was conducted by Dr Milbank Johnson and a team of scientists. He took 16 terminally ill cancer patients and subjected them to frequencies suggested by Rife for 90 days. Fourteen of the patients were cured of cancer. The remaining two took another two months to be cured.

In 1934 Rife's laboratory and his records and documents were destroyed in a suspicious fire.The AMA then labeled his work bogus and banned him. More detailed information on Rife can be found here:

Meessen, A. (2020). Virus destruction by resonance. *Journal of Modern Physics, 11*(12), 2011–2052. https://doi.org/10.4236/jmp.2020.111212 8

Even though Rife's discoveries are proven to work it is difficult to recommend the use of his technology. The problem lies in the fact that Rife's machines are expensive and there are many manufacturers. It is unknown which of these Rife machines are genuine. If you are interested in Rife, carefully research the manufacturer of the Rife device.

# 8

# Spike Proteins

S pike proteins are the bumps that protrude from the surface of viruses. These bumps change shape to match the surface of a cell. As soon as they attach themselves, they enter the cell.

Unfortunately spike proteins are present in the Pfizer and Moderna vaccines. These spike proteins turn off the genes that fight cancer, specifically the p-53 gene.This results in what is now described as Turbo-cancer. These spike proteins also clog up your vascular system resulting in Heart attacks and other heart conditions.

Today, P. (2022, November 16). VACCINE-INDUCED TURBO CANCER: T-cell lymphoma can progress rapidly due to mRNA booster shot. *Planet Today*. https://www.planet-today.com/2022/11/vaccine-induced-turbo-cancer-t-cell.html

What can you do about spike proteins?

- Spike protein inhibitors and neutralizers pine needles, Ivermectin, Neem, N-acetylcysteine (NAC) and Glutathione.

- Spike protein detox essentials vitamin D, vitamin C, nigella seed, Quercetin, zinc, curcumin, milk thistle extract, NAC, Ivermectin and magnesium.

Also, Dr. McCullough recommends three over-the-counter natural substances to degrade harmful spike proteins and reduce inflammation:

Nattokinase: 2000 fibrin units (100 milligrams) twice a day

Bromelain: 500 milligrams once a day

Curcumin: 500 milligrams twice a day (nano, liposomal, or with piperine additive suggested)

Research the dosages necessary for your particular circumstance.

# 9

# Diet Change

One of the most comprehensive studies on Nutrition and Cancer is The China Study by T. Colin Campbell PhD. This 20-year study collected data from 880 million Chinese and determined that cancer tumors grew if protein intake exceeded 10 percent. It also showed that plant protein was better than animal protein in terms of heart disease. Dr. Campbell says, "From our extensive research, one idea seemed to be clear: lower protein intake dramatically decreased tumor initiation."

Team, C. T. (2020, April 6). *The China study: The most comprehensive study of nutrition ever conducted*. Cancer Tutor. https://www.cancertuto r.com/china-study/

The China Study does not advocate a vegetarian diet. It just says to minimize protein intake below 10 percent. Though he does say plant protein is better than animal protein. He advocates the use of Vitamin D if you cannot get regular exposure to sunlight. The form of Vitamin D you should take is D3.Large doses of D3 are not dangerous. Consider that sunbathing for 30 minutes produces 20,000 IU of Vitamin D3 in your skin. Do not neglect Vitamin D3. It is an important supplement for your health.

# 10

# Fasting

There are many benefits of fasting besides saving money on food!

1. Reduces insulin resistance.

I was diagnosed many years ago with Diabetes. The doctors prescribed many different assorted drugs to control sugar. None of them worked. I decided to fast. It wasn't easy. But I persisted and now my sugar levels are normal. Please be extra careful if you are diabetic and try fasting. Do your research. Consult your Doctor.

1. Helps cardiovascular system.

Losing weight benefits your heart. Reduces your blood pressure and helps combat edema. It's that simple.

1. Reduces inflammation.

Studies have shown that intermittent fasting reduces the protein markers indicating inflammation.Inflammation shows up in many diseases.I have used fasting to help eliminate gout. For Gout I used fasting, Turmeric with black pepper and Boswellia.

1.  Improves brain function.

Studies have shown fasting increases the generation of nerve cells and helps prevent neurodegenerative diseases like Alzheimer's and Parkinsons.

1.  Extends lifespan.

Fasting increased the helpful bacteria in the gut associated with longevity Christencenella. Proteins related to longevity such as curtains were increased.

1.  Prevents cancer.

Sugar feeds cancer cells. Remove sugar by fasting and cancer stops growing.

1.  Helps weight loss.

Studies have shown fasting induces weight loss better than calorie restriction and even exercise. Up to a 9 percent reduction has been shown.

Fasting is not easy to do, if you have never tried fasting you should start slowly. Start with intermittent fasting. If you haven't eaten overnight for 12 hours you are already doing intermittent fasting.Extend your fast to longer periods of time, make sure to keep hydrated. Stop immediately if you feel dizzy or ill. For more detailed information on fasting see the link below:

Rd, H. W. (2023, May 9). *How to fast Safely: 10 helpful tips*. Healthline. https://www.healthline.com/nutrition/how-to-fast#TOC_TITLE_H DR_12

Personally, I have fasted for 10 days without any problems.

## 11

# Liver Cirrhosis

About 9 years ago I received a phone call from a Physician's assistant. The Doctor himself couldn't be bothered. She told me I had Stage III Cirrhosis of the liver determined by the sonogram of my liver.

"Oh," I said, "What's that, how do I fix it?" She paused, "It's incurable," she said. She wanted me to come in, I said ok and made an appointment. I looked up Stage III Cirrhosis of the liver and it basically said my lifespan was now 4 to 6 years maximum. That was quite disturbing.

At the appointment she wanted me to get a liver biopsy, and be put on the liver transplant list. She also advocated that I try a new treatment in a drug trial. I asked her if there were any issues with doing a liver biopsy. She said there was a 30 percent chance of complications, and I would be hospitalized for about a week. I asked her if she ever gambled or played scratch off cards. If she understood what 30 percent odds meant.No response. I then asked her what the biopsy would show. It would show if you had liver cancer. Is that curable? No, she said. Ridiculous, why would I want to know I had an incurable disease, I directly refused the biopsy. They wanted my kidney Doctor to agree to the liver drug trial. He just ignored them, looking for a scapegoat he told me.

How did I survive Stage III Liver Cirrhosis?
   I did several things:

1. Fasting, this was explained previously above
2. R-Alpha Lipoic acid, the R form is biologically active and has antioxidant properties. Reduces liver fibrosis and reverses liver damage. R-Alpha Lipoic acid 250mg twice a day.
3. Selenium detoxifies liver enzymes, reverses liver damage. Selenomethionine 200 mcg twice per day
4. Milk Thistle (Silymarin/ Silybum), antifibrotic, enhances protein production, removes toxins,heals kidney disease. Milk Thistle Seed Extract 450 mg twice per day.

12

## Pain

Over twenty-five years ago I suffered a herniated disc due to a car accident. I still remember this clearly. I was driving a Toyota Camry and was stuck in stop and go traffic on the West Side Highway in New York City heading to The Bronx.

I had a strange premonition something was about to happen, and I looked in the rear view mirror. I saw the driver behind me looking over her shoulder to her right and without looking forward again sped her car into the right lane. She didn't make it. She struck my car on the rear right. The impact was so great it shoved my car into the car in front and my car seat collapsed backward and I ended up in a flat position with my foot still on the brake.

Only 45 minutes later did I feel a pain in my lower back on the right side just above my hip. I went to a doctor and he had me get an MRI. The results indicated that I had a herniated disc between S1 and S2.

Days later the real pain kicked in, I can only describe it as if a red-hot knitting needle had been shoved into my back. This pain occurred at random times, it didn't matter if I was walking, standing, sitting or lying down. It was driving me insane.

I went back to the Doctor and asked him for a solution to this pain. I will never forget what he said, "Welcome to the rest of your life!" I remember thinking, "This Jackass thinks this is a cartoon!" That started my journey into the world of Alternative Medicine.

How did I cure my herniated disc?

Homeopathy.

At that time in my life I was learning Tai Chi from Lawrence Gallante: https://www.amazon.com/Tai-Chi-Ultimate-Lawrence-Galante/dp/0877284970

He was also a homeopathic doctor. I described my problem and asked him for a solution. "Nerve damage," he said, "take Hypericum."

I drove off to the drugstore. At this time in New York City there was only one drugstore in Manhattan that sold homeopathic remedies on 18th street. I left my friend Donald in the car, double parked and went inside. There was only one small shelf in the entire drug store and only one vial of Hypericum with the unheard-of strength of 1M for $6. I had no choice but to buy it and I drove away.

I was stopped at a red light by Washington Square Park (notorious drug den in those days) near NYU when the pain hit me.The light turned green, and I was fumbling with the vial and the steering wheel as the car moved forward. I threw 3 sugar pills in my mouth and boom the pain went away. The car had not even reached the next light. I was so shocked I started pounding myself on the back to restart the pain hoping it wasn't temporary and it wasn't, the pain was gone forever.

Homeopathy is a vast topic. Decried as Quackery in the US and hailed as a wonder medicine in Europe. The founder of Homeopathy was Samuel Hanneman. The story is that one day as he was observing mountain goats he noticed when they fell, which was very rare, they would run to a certain plant and eat it. They would then bound away as if nothing had happened. Curious, he collected samples of this plant which was called Arnica Montana and ate it himself. Bruises formed on his body and he felt aches and pain.He then postulated, "Similar cures similar." He achieved fame during the Napoleonic wars by curing troops of Dysentery. I have used Arnica after I have fallen badly and walked away unscathed.

Sciatic nerve pain

Several years ago, I developed a very bad sciatic pain running down my leg from my back. It got so bad I would flinch every time I put my foot on a stair. I remember that I had seen a device for sale on Amazon called the Deka-Titan that claimed to block nerve pain. But unfortunately, when I looked for it was no longer available. I searched my last resort website eBay and incredibly there was one for sale. I immediately bought it. It looks like a wrist watch meant to be worn on the wrist.

When I got it, I put it on and within 10 seconds my sciatic nerve pain disappeared and has never returned. I wear it all the time now just in case. I did some more research and found that it also eliminates migraine headaches. You can find the Deka-Titan on the Internet.

The Curtis technique

This technique works 95 percent of the time, works immediately and is permanent. To find the Curtis spot start in the armpit and go down about 4 inches to feel for the sore spot. This is going to be very painful.

Press into that sore spot and imagine spreading the ribs in that area. This is best understood by watching the following video.

https://www.youtube.com/watch?v=g1wBTgW6aEM

# 13

# DMSO

DMSO is extracted from trees. Trees use it to carry nutrients and to stop the trees from freezing in cold weather. It was discovered by Alexander Saytzeff in 1866. DSMO can instantly carry whatever it is mixed with throughout your body. This allows it to be combined with many herbal remedies. The use of DMSO in treating ailments is a vast topic. I can only list a few here.

- Back Pain
- Blood pressure
- Liver cirrhosis
- Alzheimer's

For more information on the use of DMSO I recommend the following book:

DMSO Dimethyl sulfoxide for Humans: Recipes &
Treatment by Herb Richards

39

# 14

# Addiction

You are addicted to drugs, cigarettes, or alcohol.Ibogaine is your solution. Some addicts were free from addiction within one day after using Ibogaine from just one treatment and stayed free from addiction.

Noller, G., Frampton, C., & Yazar-Klosinski, B. (2017). Ibogaine treatment outcomes for opioid dependence from a twelve-month follow-up observational study. *The American Journal of Drug and Alcohol Abuse, 44*(1), 37–46. https://doi.org/10.1080/00952990.2017.1310218

What is Ibogaine?

Ibogaine is one of the alkaloids found in African shrubs such as Tabernanthe iboga, Voacanga africana, and Tabernaemontana undulata.

Unfortunately, The United States Drug Enforcement Administration lists Ibogaine as a controlled substance. Currently, New Zealand has not banned its use.

# 15

# Other Diseases and Solutions

**A**rthritis, Arthrosis, Osteoporosis

Boron has been called the miracle cure. It is a mineral, when combined with oxygen it is called Borax. Boron affects bone density, the absorption of minerals such as magnesium and calcium.Assists in the body's production of Vitamin D. Supports brain function, lack of Boron leads to lack of concentration and decrease in motor skills. Dosage depends upon your circumstances. You cannot overdose on Boron but always use moderation and caution.

**Downs Syndrome Birth Defect**

It has been shown that supplying the mother with 90 essential nutrients especially zinc with the fetus less than two months old will resolve Downs Syndrome. The baby will be normal at birth. In case you are wondering what are the 90 essential minerals:

https://thewallachrevolution.com/90-essential-nutrients/

**Heart and Edema**

In Edema water is extracellular, it is not penetrating the bi-layered membrane of the cell. It needs help penetrating the membrane to hydrate the cell. Celtic salt gives that help; it has 82 minerals.It has three forms of magnesium, magnesium Sulfate, magnesium chloride and magnesium bromide. Magnesium is a water hungry mineral and helps hold all the other minerals in suspension. Magnesium helps pull the water into the cell.

Hawthorn Berry strengthens the heart. If blood pressure is high, it will lower it and if the blood pressure is low it will raise it. It is also used for inflammation.

Cayenne pepper moves the blood. It also thins the blood. It can replace blood thinners like warfarin. It rebuilds the heart muscle.

## Teeth and Gums

Comfrey contains a nutrient called Allantoin that is a wound healing nutrient. Comfrey has been used to heal bones, scars and gums for many years. Simply use comfrey as a mouthwash. Cloves can be used to prevent cavities. Research is being done to regrow teeth:

Bello, C. (2023, October 10). Scientists develop a groundbreaking new drug that makes your teeth regrow. *Euronews*. https://www.euronews.com/health/2023/08/05/a-drug-that-makes-teeth-regrow-scientists-move-closer-to-clinical-trials

A device has already been invented and marketed to regrow teeth. It uses ultrasound and you can find it here:
https://aevosystem.com/

## Red Light Therapy

Red light is visible to the naked eye. Its wavelength is between 600 - 700 nanometers.Near-infrared light's wavelength is between 700 - 1000 nanometers. The human eye sees wavelengths below 700 nm and above 400 nm. Red light therapy is approved by the FDA to treat acne, hair loss, muscle and joint pain, arthritis and blood circulation. The list of what it also heals is a long one including, glaucoma, obesity, stroke, wounds, regenerate tissue, depression, addiction, arthritis. The list is almost endless. Research papers on Red light therapy number in the tens of thousands.

## Methylene Blue

Methylene Blue was discovered in 1876 by Heinrich Caro.In 1891 it was discovered that Methylene Blue inhibited malaria parasites. It was discovered that it can help mitochondria in cellular respiration. Methylene Blue has been discovered to potentially be used in treatments for Alzheimer's and Parkinsons.It turns out that if you combine Red light therapy with Methylene blue there is a synergistic effect, there is a boost to the benefits. There are side effects with Methylene blue, please be careful with dosage.

## Hair Growth

You have read that Red light therapy can regrow hair. It also turns out Magnesium oil will also regrow hair and it's much cheaper. Magnesium is an essential mineral and most people are deficient in it. When you have diabetes and other ailments the body consumes magnesium at an accelerated rate. Yet if you consume magnesium orally over 90 percent of it will be flushed down the toilet.

The answer is to use magnesium oil on your skin. The skin absorbs magnesium easily. Many years ago, I looked in the mirror one day and noticed I was losing hair. I realized that my maternal grandfather had male pattern baldness. Everything I read said that male pattern baldness was hereditary. Well, I put magnesium oil on my head and three months later I had no baldness. My friend has hair whiter than an unused shoe brush.He soaked his feet in magnesium oil and the roots of his hair turned black. Another person I know lost her eyebrows, she took her finger, dipped it in magnesium oil and drew eyebrows on her forehead. Her eyebrows grew back where she had put magnesium oil.

# 16

# Prayer

On a final note, whenever I was in the midst of agony or close to death's door I would pray. Every time, a solution would present itself. Your will can change your body. As you have seen, your body is more than just chemicals. It resonates with frequencies; it is healed by light.

Your body renews itself over time. Your skeleton for example takes ten years to renew itself. I hope that I have shown you solutions to problems or have at least ignited your interest in learning more. There is more, so much more!

# Resources

Admin, Admin, & Admin. (2021, December 6). *Influence of church bells on human health.* Orthodox Christian Tools/Store/Blog- Best Answers to Your Spiritual Questions - Answers to Your Spiritual Health Questions! https://orthochristiantoo ls.com/influence-of-church-bells-on-human-health/

Bello, C. (2023, October 10). Scientists develop a groundbreaking new drug that makes your teeth regrow. *Euronews.* https://www.euron ews.com/health/2023/08/05/a-drug-that-makes-teeth-regrow-scienti sts-move-closer-to-clinical-trials

*C8 Science Panel website.* (n.d.). http://www.c8sciencepanel.org/

Costas-Ferreira, C., Durán, R., & Faro, L. (2022). Toxic effects of glyphosate on the nervous system: a systematic review. *International Journal of Molecular Sciences, 23*(9), 4605. https://doi.org/10.3390/ijms 23094605

*Did a vaccine experiment on US soldiers cause the 'Spanish flu'?* - *LewRockwell.* (2020, March 30). LewRockwell. https://www.lewro ckwell.com/2020/03/no_author/did-a-vaccine-experiment-on-u-s-so ldiers-cause-the-spanish-flu/

*Dirt road discussions.* (n.d.). Telegram. https://t.me/DirtRoadDiscussi

on/6895

*EWG finds little-known toxic chemical in four out of five people tested.* (2024, February 15). Environmental Working Group. https://www.ew g.org/news-insights/news/2024/02/ewg-finds-little-known-toxic-ch emical-four-out-five-people-tested

Faarfm, K. C. D. F. (2023, February 6). Some truths behind conventional cancer therapies. *Conners Clinic | Alternative Cancer Coaching.* https://www.connersclinic.com/the-truth-behind-conventional-cance r-therapies/

*Florida State Surgeon General calls for halt in the use of COVID-19 mRNA vaccines | Florida Department of Health.* (2024, January 20). https://www. floridahealth.gov/newsroom/2024/01/20240103-halt-use-covid19-m rna-vaccines.pr.html

Gaines, M. (2024, February 2). Roundup lawsuit update February 2024. *Forbes Advisor.* https://www.forbes.com/advisor/legal/product-l iability/roundup-lawsuit-update/

*Get busy living.* (n.d.). https://mycancerstory.rocks/

Meessen, A. (2020). Virus destruction by resonance. *Journal of Modern Physics, 11*(12), 2011–2052. https://doi.org/10.4236/jmp.2020.111212 8

Miaomt, J. K. D. (2023). Fluoride exposure and human health risks. *IAOMT.* https://iaomt.org/resources/fluoride-facts/fluoride-exposure -human-health-risks/

Millennium Products. (n.d.). *Miracle Salt.* https://millennium-produ cts.com/products/miracle-salt

Noller, G., Frampton, C., & Yazar-Klosinski, B. (2017). Ibogaine treatment outcomes for opioid dependence from a twelve-month follow-up observational study. *The American Journal of Drug and Alcohol Abuse, 44*(1), 37–46. https://doi.org/10.1080/00952990.2017.1310218

*Parasite cleanse: DIY protocol, pills, and home remedy.* (n.d.). The Berkeley Well-Being Institute. https://www.berkeleywellbeing.com/p

arasite-cleanse-protocol-pills-home-remedy.html

Phillips, K. (2020, July 27). Herxheimer reaction - Feeling worse before feeling better. *Colloidal Silver | Silver Colloids*. https://www.silver-colloids.com/herxheimer-reaction/

Raccioppi, R. M. (2014, March 10). 528Hz - DNA repair - art and science of restorative frequencies. *Nyack-Piermont, NY Patch*. https://patch.com/new-york/nyack/528hz—dna-repair—art-and-science-of-restorative-frequencies

Rd, H. W. (2023, May 9). *How to fast Safely: 10 helpful tips*. Healthline. https://www.healthline.com/nutrition/how-to-fast#TOC_TITLE_HDR_12

Science, E. O. G. (2020, October 28). *Fake peer-reviewing*. The Embassy of Good Science. https://embassy.science/wiki/Theme:Fb1a2e2a-aa2a-4eb4-ac9c-c9567c2b401b

Selby, K., RN. (2023, December 20). *High cost of cancer treatment: chemotherapy & other options*. Mesothelioma Center - Vital Services for Cancer Patients & Families. https://www.asbestos.com/featured-stories/high-cost-of-cancer-treatment/

Team, C. T. (2020, April 6). *The China study: The most comprehensive study of nutrition ever conducted*. Cancer Tutor. https://www.cancertutor.com/china-study/

Team, S. L. (2024, February 6). *Are you snacking on Cancer-Causing weed killer? Here are the foods you need to avoid*. Sokolove Law. https://www.sokolovelaw.com/blog/foods-glyphosate-cancer/

Thomas, S. P. (2018). Current controversies regarding peer review in scholarly journals. *Issues in Mental Health Nursing, 39*(2), 99–101. https://doi.org/10.1080/01612840.2018.1431443

Timshina, A., Aristizabal-Henao, J. J., Da Silva, B. F., & Bowden, J. A. (2021). The last straw: Characterization of per- and polyfluoroalkyl substances in commercially-available plant-based drinking straws. *Chemosphere, 277*, 130238. https://doi.org/10.1016/j.chemosphere.

2021.130238

Today, P. (2022, November 16). VACCINE-INDUCED TURBO CANCER: T-cell lymphoma can progress rapidly due to mRNA booster shot. *Planet Today*. https://www.planet-today.com/2022/11/vaccine-induced-turbo-cancer-t-cell.html

Wilson, R. (2023, September 1). *Childhood Vaccines cause Autism: The evidence and the institutional cover-up.* The Expose. https://expose-news.com/2023/09/01/childhood-vaccines-cause-autism-the-evidence-and-the-institutional-cover-up/

Yeager, A. (2011, November 15). *A sip or quick dip could change your DNA - Research Blog.* Research Blog. https://researchblog.duke.edu/2011/11/15/a-sip-or-quick-dip-could-change-your-dna/